A
For
ght
Loss

YOGA
For
Weight
Loss

Bharat Thakur

wisdom
tree

— To my parents

Copyright © 2003, Bharat Thakur
Reprinted March 2003; July 2003

ISBN 81-86685-31-6

Cover Picture Courtsey: Tarun Khewal

Cover Design: Kamal P. Jammual

Published by

Wisdom Tree
C-209/1 Mayapuri, Phase-II,
New Delhi-110 064.
Tel.: 28111720, 28114437

Printed at

Print Perfect,
New Delhi-110 064.

Preface

I was walking around in the marketplace when the idea to write a book on 'Yoga for Weight Loss' came into my head. Eighty per cent of the people I saw there, were either obese or overweight. Though I am here to spread my guru's teachings and make human lives better and enlightened, I wondered why I was preaching enlightenment when men cannot even look into the mirror and ask, "What have I done to myself?" Yes, what have you done to yourself? You will die without knowing that you can look amazing! That hidden inside your sick, fat and obese body, lies somebody who is healthy and fit and loves himself.

Wake up! Stop feeling jealous of people who have an amazing physique and body structure! Instead, fix yourself and become that! You complain that your girlfriend sitting beside you is looking at another man with such wonder in her eyes or that your husband's gaze keeps straying to beautiful women, when all you need to do is take your body in your own hands and be that person.

Just look at yourself — take a long, hard look. What do you see? Your stomach — so huge! Your butt — so big! But most men and women in India (or else where) are like this, you will say. This is a mere consolation and you know very well that you are not confronting the real issue. Make friends with people who are fitness freaks and let them make you feel low because of their confidence and beauty. Understand that you too could be beautiful if you stopped being an escapist. Have the courage to challenge yourself with the conviction that you are the most intelligent and conscious creature of all species on this planet! And then live up to it! Use your intellect that is innocent of any pre-conceptions to question your present state. All you need to do is simply come to a decision that yes, I will!

www.bharatthakur.com

Contents

Understanding Obesity

Obesity is essentially a state of metabolic disturbance. It happens when there is an imbalance between the intake and expenditure of energy in the body. Despite a growing awareness on the dangers of obesity, it is increasing at an alarming rate. The primary causes of this are the marked changes in culture and lifestyle.

In the present scenario, there is a discernible shift in the focus of life. Growing material needs now take a greater priority over pursuit of happiness. Things really changed during the industrial revolution. Machines took over from man and though they hastened the rate of work, man became physically lazy in the process. This is the predominant cause of the dismal state of our bodies. Undoubtedly, obesity is a curse.

There are two types of obesity — chronic and fluctuating. Most overweight people usually fall into the category of fluctuating obesity since they tend to gain and lose weight at different times. In the chronic condition, the person is severely overweight and tends to gain more and more weight with time. To help an overweight person lose weight is easy. But an obese person has to work harder as his system has become used to the excessive weight.

All I ask an obese or overweight person is just one thing: a strong determination to say, "No" to a life of excess weight. Just one pledge that, "From today, I decide to change my life in every possible way to get my body in shape and lead a healthy and happy life."

Definition of Obesity

Obesity, according to me, is a mental state of lethargy and depression leading to an imbalance between energy intake and output, thus leading to excessive weight on the whole body or in a localised area.

Obesity takes on various forms depending upon the nature of fat-deposition in the body:

- *Harmonious Obesity*: In such cases, the fat is distributed all over the body

- *Gynoid Obesity*: In such cases, the fat deposits are more on the lower part of the body— the hip and the pelvic area. This is more prominent in women and carriers the lowest medical risk.

- *Visceral Obesity*: In such cases, the fat is deposited near the internal organs such as the abdomin visceres. This fat is not apparent from outside and carries the highest long-term medical risks.

- *Android Obesity*: In such cases, the fat deposition is more on the external stomach area. It is more prominent in males and is generally dangerous.

Measuring Obesity

Every culture has its own standards of beauty. What is considered obese in one culture might be normal in another. So, there is no absolute and fixed indicator of obesity. However, a comparison of weight to height can give us a good idea of how obese the person is. The BMI (Body Mass Index) is used widely for the purpose of measuring obesity. It is calculated by dividing the weight (in kilograms) by the square of height (in metres). This measures applies to both men and women.

The formula for estimating BMI is given below:

$$BMI = \frac{\text{weight (in kgs)}}{\text{height x height (in metres)}}$$

While converting height from FPS to SI system the following conversion equations are used:

1 Foot = 12 inches
1 Inch = 2.54 cms
1 m   = 100 cms

For example, a man 5' 7" (67 inches or 1.7 metres), weighing 82 kgs, has a BMI of

$$\frac{82}{1.7 \text{ x } 1.7} = 28.3 \text{ kg/m}^2$$

To get a measure of obesity, we use the following scale:

- A BMI between 19 to 25 kg/m^2 indicates normal or optimum weight.
- A BMI between 25 to 30 kg/m^2 indicates overweight.
- A BMI between 30 to 35 kg/m^2 indicates obesity.
- A BMI above 35 kg/m^2 indicates gross obesity.

According to the scale given above, this man is overweight.

It is interesting to know that in hunting – gathering cultures (like the Bushmen of the Kalahari and the Australian Aborigines), the BMI's are far below 18 kg/m^2. These people do not have problems like heart diseases, high blood pressure or diabetes. This level of BMI is impossible and unnecessary for most people to reach. The medically accepted ideal BMI (19 to 25 kg/m^2) should be the target for every overweight or obese person.

How Obesity Happens

The weight of an individual is a result of many factors. It is the outcome of a complex relationship between the physiological, genetic and psychological constitution, environmental and cultural factors, lifestyle and of course, eating habits of the individual. Besides, an individual body reacts differently to different situations. Some people can eat too much of food, not exercise and still not gain any weight. Others may eat little but still tend to put on weight easily. Emotional problems

4

like depression, loneliness and trauma can lead to sudden weight gain because people tend to overeat in such situations. Dieting can also lead to obesity as most dieters try to grow thinner by drastically cutting down the food intake. This eventually leads to 'binge eating' and a further increase in weight. Malfunctioning of the thyroid or the pituitary glands can also lead to obesity. When a person has obese parents, he or she is at a higher risk of being obese. So we see that all these factors, operating by themselves or in conjunction with each other, can lead to obesity.

The human body has an amazing mechanism in form of the hypothalamus, situated in the centre of the brain. This gland regulates feelings of hunger and satiety. It tells you when you are hungry so that you can eat and then tells you when you are full, so that you can stop. It sends messages via certain hormones called neurotransmitters that either stimulate or inhibit hunger. These neurotransmitters are Adrenalin, Noradrenalin, Dopamine and Serotonine. There are also other drugs like Anorexigines and Flemfluramines that act on these neurotransmitters and control their release so that there is a perfect regulation of a person's appetite according to the energy output and intake.

The human body also has another complex and amazing weight regulating mechanism by which it can use stored fat when there is little or no energy intake in form of food. Weight loss diets are based on this principle but this alone never works in the long term. The body must never be deprived of the nutrients and energy that it genuinely requires.

Let us now look at how the body expends it's energy. Basically, the body expends energy in three ways:

- *Metabolism*: This is the minimum energy needed for the body to remain alive. It accounts for 70 per cent of the total energy output. It also depends on the muscles (lean mass) of a person. People with high BMR (Basic Metabolic Rates) will consume more calories and also use them up as easily.

- *Physical Activity*: This accounts for 20 per cent of the output but varies from person-to-person depending on the level of activity. Obese people require more calories for performing the same activity because they carry excess weight. Thus, they tend to eat more to compensate for this, leading to a vicious cycle.

- *Thermogenesis*: This accounts for about 10 per cent of the total output and it is the energy used during the digestive process itself. Because of this, some calories absorbed during a meal are expended immediately. Skipping a meal is therefore not advisable.

Energy intake refers to the quantity of food, quality of food and the eating habits of a person. A manual labourer uses up more energy as compared to a software engineer so he will tend to eat more food. Quality of food refers to the ratio of nutrients in the food eaten. Too much fat, sugar or refined food in the diet, leads to obesity. Other good food habits include regular eating hours and not skipping meals.

So at the physiological level, the body tends to gain weight when there is an imbalance between energy taken in and the energy released because of the factors mentioned above. To lose weight and not put it back, the body has to be trained to regain this balance once again. This is the challenge that faces every obese or overweight person.

Health Risks of Obesity

Obesity is associated with many health risks. And like the causes of obesity, these risks are often related to one another. The common risks are:

- *High Blood Pressure*: Obese people are approximately twice as likely to have high blood pressure than people with a normal BMI range between 19 and 25. High blood pressure may lead to stroke and heart diseases.
- *Diabetes*: Obesity significantly increases the risk of Type 2 Diabetes, where the body is unable to produce enough Insulin or use it properly. Men with fat accumulation in the abdomen area are specifically under risk.
- *Coronary Heart Disease*: Obesity leads to higher levels of cholesterol and high blood pressure which are both directly related to cardiovascular risks.
- *Gall Bladder Disease*: Obesity has a direct correlation with this disease in both men and women. However, women have a greater risk of developing gall bladder problems as compared to men.
- *Arthritis*: Obese women are at a greater risk of arthritis and joint pain as compared to men.

- *Cancer:* Obese men are at a greater risk of developing colon cancer, whereas obese women are at risk of developing breast cancer and cancer of the uterus.
- *Breathing Problems:* Obese people have difficulty in breathing enough air so their oxygen intake is low.
- *Premature Death:* Obese people tend to die sooner than those with normal weight.

There are enough reasons why an obese person should tackle this disease and break out from the vicious cycle where his or her mental state initially leads to weight gain and this in turn, leads to further weight gain. A person has to work hard at the physiological level as well as the psychological level, to permanently get rid of this disease. And if you make a firm decision within yourself, nothing can stop you.

2

Yoga And Weight Loss

The word Yoga originates from the Sanskrit word, *Yuj* which means union— union of the self with the universal consciousness. This book will deal with obesity as a disease and will help a layman understand the entire psychology, physiology and other related details on the issue. Yoga is not just the physical practice of *asanas*, nor is it a spiritual philosophy or religion. It is the means to become an ideal human being. It works from the body to the breath and from the breath to the mind and later, to the super-consciousness. Yoga is the ultimate truth. It takes man from a raw state of consciousness to an enlightened one.

Let us look at the connection between Yoga and obesity — a disease/ state of mind. In the past, Yoga had a different approach— it was a serious spiritual journey. This is evident from ancient texts like *Ghirand Samhita, Hatha Pradeepika* and *Vashishta Yoga*. With time, research revealed the medical benefits of Yoga. Gradually, it took the status of alternative medicine as it was able to cure many diseases which modern science has not been able to fathom. Yoga has an immense understanding of the mind, body and to a great extent, that which lies beyond. This, Yoga calls the *chitta* or consciousness.

Yoga has evolved from the trials and tribulations of *yogis* in different states of health, moods and disease, in their endeavour towards achieving what lay beyond the body. Every *asana* was a copy of an animal's posture. The *yogis* looked, observed, analysed and started performing them as a means to heal themselves. In the process, they went beyond healing and cured the cause of the disease itself. Therefore, Yoga does not treat obesity only by considering it a disease or a disturbed mental state. It addresses the causes and the possibilities by which the body can be brought to a state of ideal functioning.

Yoga works in a unique manner. It does not believe in burning calories and draining the body energy but tries to work on the endocrinal system and change the hormonal balance in the body. This in turn, changes the *pH* of the blood and tones up the muscles. Physiologically, Yoga works on the concept of stretching and applying pressure on the endocrinal glands. Unwanted fat from the body is removed by burning calories as well as by altering the hormonal balance of the whole body. Thus the homeostasis (internal environment) of the body also changes. Yogic *asanas* tone up the body by penetrating deep into each tissue and muscle which general exercises cannot achieve. *Asanas* are postures that stretch all the *nadis* of the body. As per the *Gherand Samhita*, there are 72,000 *nadis* in the body.

Yoga tries to understand the root cause of any functional disorder in the body. Yoga says that 90 per cent of functional disorders are because of a lack of understanding of the human body, clarity and purpose in life and lack of awareness. This takes the body into a state of *vikshipta chitta* (diseased state of mind). I firmly believe that to cure a problem like obesity, one has to look into one's personal life, personal habits and the reasons for existence. We are all here to become a Buddha but instead, we end up living in depression and develop wrong habits. Of course, there are medical causes responsible for obesity as in case of Thyroid related problems, where one has to take harmful drugs like steroids that directly raise the appetite and increase food consumption, thus indirectly altering the homeostasis of the body.

We will deal with weight loss by first trying to understand the causes of obesity. And then, we shall proceed to build mental power, change eating habits, with the practice of Yoga as the basis. This will hasten the process of curing obesity. Yoga is not against activities like jogging, walking, swimming or working out in the gym. I encourage all these activities. If you can jog or swim for half an hour every day besides practicing Yoga, you will lose weight at an even faster rate. Practicing Yoga will help your muscles stay flexible, supple and firm and the practice of *kapalbhati kriya*, for example, will help you jog for longer periods of time as it helps cardiovascular endurance. Yoga affects all aspects of the body — cardiovascular, hormonal and muscular. You will find that your performance in every single activity will improve significantly with the practice of Yoga. Breathing exercises (*pranayama*) which are a form of meditation, will help you understand life from a broader perspective, shift the focus of your life, rectify wrong habits and show you how to go beyond your indulgences. Yoga is essential if you want to change the functioning of your entire system, lose weight, build a healthy muscle tone and live a healthy lifestyle where gaining weight becomes practically impossible.

3

Essentials of Yogic Practices

What is an Asana?

Patanjali's *Yoga Sutras* define *asanas* as *"sthiraha sukham asanam."* Translated, it means stability, feeling of well-being and a posture. So *asanas* are those postures that give a feeling of well-being and stability. There are 84 lakh postures in Yoga and all of them basically target to prepare a person for just four postures – *siddhasana*, *padmasana*, *vajrasana* and *sukhsasana*. All these are meditative postures. So one should perform all these postures with the aim of being able to maintain them for a long duration. Yoga starts from *yama* and *niyama* and ends at *samadhi*.

How to Perform Asanas

Patanjali says, *"prayatna saithilyam anantha samap prathibyan."* Translated, this means, one should try to perform a posture effortlessly by fixing the mind beyond. Here, 'beyond' implies the plane above all mundane concerns of life. One should be aware only of things like breath, music, movement from one posture to another or the target muscle that is stretched in the posture.

Benefits

Patanjali says, *"twato dwandad nabhi ghatah."* Translated, this means that on the performance of *asanas*, one can be free from all dualities in life. Here, 'duality' symbolises a lack of clarity and vision in life.

Discipline

Patanjali says, *"atha yoga nushasanam."* Translated, this means, the discipline of Yoga. Patanjali meant that, before you enter the realm of Yoga, you have to learn to be aware of the fact that you cannot perform *yogic* practices without being totally focused on the present moment.

Place

One should try to practice Yoga in an open space if possible. But in today's scenario of high pollution levels, it is not safe to practice *yogic* breathing while inhaling toxins like carbon monoxide which hurt the system. If you live in a polluted metropolitan city, I would advise you to practice Yoga in a nice and clean room.

Duration

There are two aspects to duration in Yoga. One is the total duration for the performance of Yoga and the second is the duration for each *asana*. One can practice Yoga for twenty minutes, forty minutes or five hours a day. This depends on what is desired from Yoga. If the need is basic flexibility of the body and stress-relief, one can be benefited in just twenty minutes. If one wants enlightenment, five hours are also not enough. As far as the duration of maintaining a posture is concerned, one could start with ten seconds and increase this upto thirty seconds or a minute.

Equipments

There are no specific equipments required as such for the practice of Yoga. However, one can use ropes, bricks, round pillows, elastic belts, and of course, the Yoga mat.

Atmosphere

A hygenic and serene atmosphere is very important for the practice of Yoga. It could be an open space, a beautiful site or a nice clean room with gentle lighting.

Fragrance

You should try to practice Yoga where there is plenty of natural fragrance around. Flowers, plants, trees, soil etc., all have their own aroma. If you practice Yoga in a room, you should always light an incense stick or an aromatic candle. This will make you feel more relaxed and focused.

Music

As mentioned earlier, maintaining a posture and fixing the mind 'beyond' is the technique for performing *asanas*. For this, nothing could be better than natural surroundings — the music of chirping birds or the movement of trees. You can also listen to devotional music and if you appreciate Indian classical music, then *ragas* can be played.

Repetition

Yoga does not believe in repeating a posture but maintaining each posture for as long as possible. But if you cannot maintain a posture for long because of lack of strength, you can perform each posture twice or thrice till you gain strength to perform it for a longer duration.

Breathing

Breathing right is very important for the practice of Yoga. A simple rule to follow is to inhale when you bend backwards and exhale while bending forwards. Whenever you perform a posture, breathe normally, except when indicated otherwise.

Pace

The pace of changing *yogic* postures except for *surya namaskar*, should be very slow and performed in steps. To move from one basic posture into another, within the same *asana*, is an *asana* in itself.

Time Between Food and Yoga

One should not perform difficult or intense *yogic* postures soon after lunch or dinner. A minimum gap of an hour after heavy meals and half-an-hour after breakfast is recommended. It is advisable to practice Yoga on an empty stomach for best results.

Clothes

One should wear clothes that allow plenty of freedom of movement in all directions. These could vary from being skin-tight to very loose as per personal convenience.

Regularity

One has to be very regular with *yogic* practices as muscles and joints take a lot of time to become flexible. Practicing for four days and missing one day means going back to square one. Therein lies the importance of regularity.

Combination of Asanas

To support the right posture, two muscle groups called the antagonist and the agonist work together. When you curl the hands at the elbows, the biceps become the agonist and the triceps become the antagonist. One should know that *asanas* should be performed for both the muscle groups. If you perform a forward-bending posture, it should be followed by a backward-bending posture. For a complete hourly Yoga workout, you should select postures for every part of the body. These include sitting, standing, supine line (lying on the back) and prone line (lying on the stomach) postures.

Order of Yogic Practices

The order in which *yogic* practices should be performed, is as follows:

1. *Pranayama*
2. *Bandha*
3. *Mudra*
4. *Kriya*
5. *Asana*

Pranayama calls for a relaxed breathing pattern. If one performs *pranayama* after *asanas*, the breathing pattern becomes faster which is not good for *pranayama sadhana* (practice). *Bandhas* are followed by *pranayama* because certain *bandhas* have to be performed along with *pranayama*. *Mudras* and *kriyas* increase the Basic Metabolic Rate (BMR) of the body which makes it easier to perform *asanas*.

Medical Problems

People with specific medical problems should consult their doctor before they perform certain *asanas*. For example, if you are a patient of high blood pressure, you should not perform *sirshasana*.

4

Pranayama

Most obese people worry about their weight. *Pranayama* helps to lower their anxiety level and improve will power. To reduce weight, one needs tremendous will power. In most weight-loss programs, people are either unable to discipline themselves to lose weight or else, they lose weight initially but are unable to maintain the program. Practicing *pranayama* is a way to start living for the moment, not get worried about how much weight you need to lose; instead, focus on your resolve to lose weight and the steps you need to take to reach your goal.

Prana means 'breath' and *ayam* means 'control'. Thus, *Pranayama* is a technique of breath control. Breathing is an amazing activity. If it stops, we die; and if we become constantly aware of it, we achieve enlightenment. It is the connecting cord between the conscious and superconscious states which can lead an individual to *moksha shareer* (the state of ultimate freedom). In his book, *Shiva Samhita*, Lord Shiva says that if one becomes aware of one's breath, the mind gets controlled and vice-versa. To control the mind, one needs to control the breath. No other religion or science has studied respiration as well as deeply as Yoga. *Pranayama* is the art of wishful awareness of the entire breathing system. It is a form of meditation. However, this wishful awareness cannot happen without being trained or conditioned in certain skills and techniques. *Yogis* have devised innumerable varieties of *pranayama* which affect different aspects of the brain and body. Some techniques work to decrease the body temperature, while others increase it, thereby altering all endocrinal (hormonal) secretions.

So what are the benefits of *pranayama*? And why should a person practice the various techniques of *pranayama* for fifteen minutes everyday? What will it achieve? To understand this, all we need to do is study our breathing pattern under different conditions: the number of breaths per minute in a sitting position — twelve to sixteen; while sleeping — thirty to thirty-five; when angry—forty-five to sixty; and two to three breaths when relaxed. The philosophy of Yoga says that a human being's age is directly related to the total number of breaths he takes in his lifetime. When a person practices certain techniques of *pranayama*, he changes his breathing pattern for the entire day. The number of breaths per minute in all the situations discussed above start getting lesser and lesser with every passing day and slowly, the person starts feeling more peaceful and relaxed. The oneness between his physical and mental body is heightened.

There are three parts of *pranayama*: *purak* (controlled inhalation), *rechak* (controlled exhalation) and *kumbhak* (retention).

Kumbhak is the most important aspect of *pranayama* and it is further sub-divided into three parts:

- *Antar kumbhak* — inhaling and holding the breath.
- *Wahiyah kumbhak* — exhaling and holding the breath.
- *Kevala kumbhak* — Surviving without air for some time. One gift of practicing *pranayama* is that man can still survive when the entire breathing system ceases. *Yogis* can even reach a level of awareness where their heart beat decreases to a minimum.

How Pranayama Works

Respiration has two effects on our body — external and internal. When one inhales, the chest moves upwards, the thoracic cage expands and the intercostal muscles of the ribs draw closer. When one exhales, the chest comes down and the intercostal muscles of the ribs get stretched. This is the external effect of respiration.

When one inhales, air enters through the nostrils and passes through the trachea to reach the lungs and the small alveoli sacs in the lungs swell-up like a balloon. Each alveoli sac is surrounded by blood vessels which exchange carbon dioxide and oxygen with the air inside. When one inhales and holds the breath, one allows enough time for the Haemoglobin (Hb) present in blood, to combine with oxygen to form Oxyhaemoglobin which enriches and energises the whole body ($Hb + O_2 = HbO_2$). *Pranayama* therefore, is the art of revitalising the whole system.

What should be the ideal ratio of *purak kumbhak* and *rechak?* Ideally speaking, the ratio should be 1 : 4 : 2. As a beginner, you should not hold the breath for a period of four times the duration of inhalation. You can start with a retention period of twice the period of inhalation. After practicing for a month or so, you can increase the retention period to three times the period of inhalation and after a practice of three months, increase this to four times the period of inhalation. For example, if one counts from one to five while inhaling, one should hold the breath till ten counts and try to exhale between eight to ten counts, as per the capacity of the lungs.

BHRAMRI PRANAYAMA

Position:

Take the posture of *padamasana* or *vajrasana*.

Technique:

- Close your eyes and inhale deeply while counting from one to five.
- Hold your breath and press your chin down on the jugular notch (the mid-point of the two collar bones under the chin).
- Raise your chin up to four fingers above the jugular notch and emit the humming sound of a bee from your throat. This sound should travel upwards and spread all over the head.
- Repeat all the three parts in a rhythmical pattern. Try and increase the period of inhalation so that you can hum for a longer period without getting tired. Do not overhold the breath, otherwise your next cycle won't be the same as the previous one.

Benefits:

- The vibrations caused by the hum perform a massage on the brain. As a result, all the constricted nerves and vessels get dilated—vaso-constriction to vaso-dialation. Some anti-stress hormones are released in the process (research under progress) which bring about a state of rest.
- All the senses come together and get focused in course of the humming. This leads to a development of concentration, memory and the higher mental faculties.
- The vocal chords in the throat get relaxed while humming. This improves the quality of voice.

Don'ts:

- People with severe throat problems should avoid this *pranayama*.

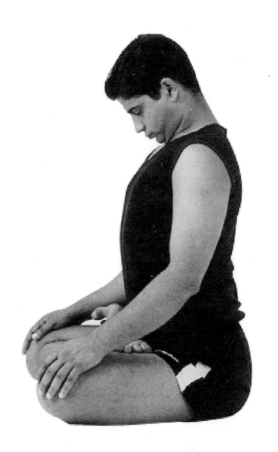

23

Sahaja Pranayama

Position:

Take the posture of *padmasana*.

Technique:

- Keep your back straight and close the eyes.
- Focus all attention on the navel region— the point of fire in the body.
- Inhale deeply, lock your chin on the jugular notch and hold your breath for as long as possible.
- Raise your chin up and exhale through the mouth.
- Repeat the three stages of this cycle in a rhythmic fashion.

Benefits:

- Holding the breath and concentrating on the navel region, increases temperature of the body and burns calories, thus helping to reduce weight.

Don'ts:

- People with cervical spondylosis should not press the chin downwards. They can keep their chin up while practicing this *pranayama*.

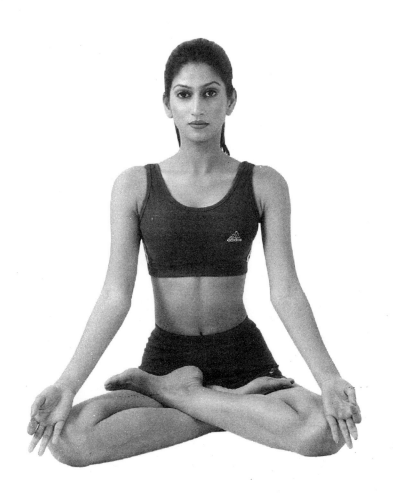

25

5

Bandha

Bandhas are neuromuscular locks that remove blockages in the glandular system of the body. Performance of *bandhas* puts pressure on the endocrinal glands and activates them. This enhances the secretion of hormones as all glands are porous in nature. Thus, the hormonal level changes in the blood stream, which helps in reducing weight.

Jalandhar Bandha

Position:

Take the posture of *padmasana* or *vajrasana*.

Technique:

- Inhale deeply, fill your lungs with air, raise your chest and hold your breath.
- Bend your chin down on the jugular notch slowly and press hard. Hold your breath for between thirty seconds to a minute.
- Raise your chin up and continue to hold your breath. When the head is back in the previous position, exhale through your nostrils.
- Repeat this cycle three times.

Benefits:

- When we press the chin down on the jugular notch, the parathyroid and the thyroid glands in the neck get activated and Thyroxin is secreted. This hormone helps in reducing stress.
- Helps in controlling diseases of the thyroid gland.

Don'ts:

- People suffering from cervical spondylosis should not perform this *bandha*, as forward bending of the neck is prohibited for them.
- This *bandha* is only for people whose Thyroxin levels are low. People with high Thyroxin levels should not perform this *bandha*.

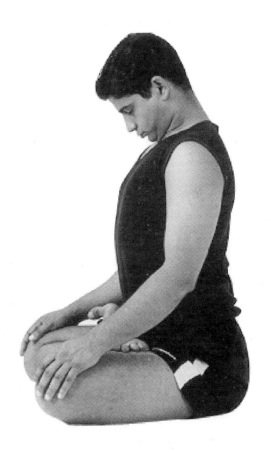

29

Mool Bandha

Position:

Take the posture of *padmasana* or *sahajasana*.

Technique:

- Exhale deeply through your mouth and hold your breath.
- Slowly squeeze your anal area (as you would, if you tried to stop passing urine). All your lower abdominal muscles should be tightly contracted.
- Release the anal area slowly and expand your abdominal muscles.
- To perform inhale slowly and relax your body.
- The *bandha* again, first take a few deep long breaths to bring your breathing back to normal.
- Repeat this cycle three times.

Benefits:

- Improves the secretion of glands situated in the lower abdominal area of the body. This increases vitality and sexual ability.

Don'ts:

- People suffering from Piles should perform this *bandha* under expert guidance.
- Women suffering from gynaecological problems should consult their doctor before performing this *bandha*.

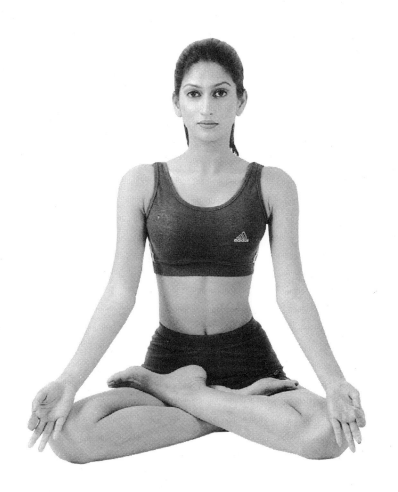

Udyaan Bandha

Position:
- Stand straight with your feet apart and parallel to the shoulders.

Technique:
- Lower your body and place your palms on your knees, thumbs outward. Exhale deeply through your mouth, hold the breath (*wahiyah kumbhak*) pull in your stomach for as long as possible.
- Get up and then inhale.
- Repeat the cycle two to three times.

Benefits:
- Research indicates that there is a pressure change of −20 to −80 mm of Hg inside the abdomen during the performance of *udyan bandha*. This triggers release of gastric juices which help in the digestive process.

Don'ts:
- People suffering from lower backache should perform this *bandha* in a sitting or standing position.
- People suffering from Asthma should not hold the breath for too long.

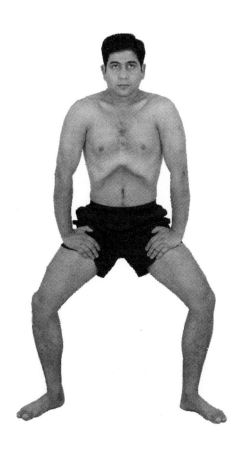

6

Kriya

Yogic *kriyas* increase the amount of oxygen consumed by the body. This affects the functioning of the heart and lungs. It speeds up the pumping of blood and deepens the breathing, thus enriching the body with oxygen. This in turn, increases the BMR (Basic Metabolic Rate) and helps in the reduction of weight.

AGNISAR KRIYA

Position:
- Stand straight with your feet spread apart and parallel to the shoulders.

Technique:
- Lower your body and place your palms on your knees, thumbs outward.
- Exhale deeply through your mouth and hold the breath (*wahiyah kumbhak*).
- Hold your breath and move your abdominal muscles in and out as many times as possible.
- Repeat this ten times and practice to increase this to between fifty and seventy cycles in one stretch.
- Get up and then inhale.
- Bring your breathing rate back to normal and relax.

Benefits:
- Improves the peristaltic movement of the stomach and helps digestion.
- Helps to remove stored stool in the stomach and consequently, control constipation.
- Strengthens the abdominal muscles and removes fat from the abdominal area.

Don'ts:
- People who have undergone Hernia or any stomach surgery should consult their doctor before performing this *kriya*.

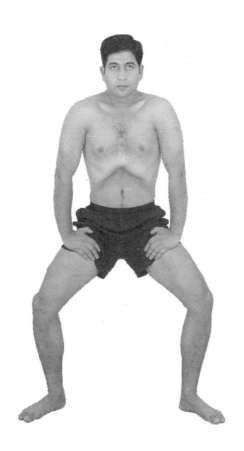

KAPALBHATI KRIYA

Kapalbhati deals with active exhalations and passive inhalations. Exhalation has immense physical and spiritual benefits, apart from providing mental relaxation. Spiritual gurus use this technique to enhance spiritual growth, particularly to activate the *kundalini* (latent power in a human being).

Position:

    Take the posture of *vajrasana* or *padmasana*.

Technique:

- Place your palms on the knees, keep the back perfectly straight and maintain a four finger gap between your chin and the jugular notch. Eyes can be kept closed. Keep the cervical area straight and try to experience the *prana* flowing throughout the spine.
- Perform forceful, powerful and active exhalations and passive inhalations in a rhythmic pattern. With every exhalation, the stomach should hit the spine or, in other words, the stomach should go inwards. Between every two exhalations, there should be an automatic inhalation which takes the stomach back to its original position.
- Start practicing with fifty exhalations at a stretch, then increase the count to a hundred. Subsequently, perform the *kriya* for two minutes continuously and increase the duration to ten minutes a day.

Benefits:

- Because of the increase of Basic Metabolic Rate during the practice of *kapalbhati kriya*, it becomes a cardiovascular exercise, thus helping weight loss. The effect of *kapalbhati* on cardiovascular endurance is phenomenal. The findings of my study done on college students

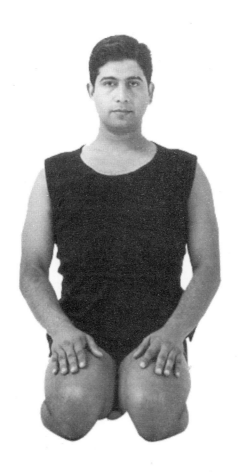

(for ten weeks) indicated that on regular performance of *kapalbhati* for fifteen minutes a day, improved the cardio-respiratory endurance. Other parameters like resting respiratory rate, pulse rate, breath-holding capacity, vital capacity (the amount of air expelled from the lungs after a deep inhalation) and cardiovascular endurance (the ability of the circulatory and respiratory system to adjust to vigorous exercise and to recover from it) were also significantly altered, indicating a higher level of fitness.

- Helps in removing excessive fat from the body by activating the peristaltic movement in the stomach. Because of the rhythmical active exhalations, the stomach moves in and out, affecting the entire alimentary canal. All sorts of toxins and unwanted stool in that area get removed.
- Changes the faulty breathing pattern of people who breathe through their mouths or snore.
- Helps cure Sinusitis, Migraine and Hypertension. Forceful exhalations enrich the body by flushing out the toxins and unwanted air from the system, increasing the amount of oxygen intake and subsequently revitalising the system.
- Helps to awaken the lowest plexus (group of nerves called the *chakra*) called the *mooladhara* and this in turn, activates the *kundalini*.

Don'ts:
- Those suffering from high blood pressure, gynaecological problems, stomach ailments, or who have undergone surgery recently should not practice this *kriya* without consulting their doctor.

7

Asana

If performed with diligence and focus, *asanas* are the key *yogic* practice for weight loss. But this calls for rigour and sustained endeavour. Each posture should be maintained for a long duration. There are two ways of ensuring this:

- Successively increasing the duration of each posture.
- Successively increasing the frequency of performing the posture.

Initially, the body will take time to adapt to the stress and strain caused by the *asanas,* so start slowly. Begin with twenty minutes a day and increase this period to an hour within three months. Different bodies react differently to Yoga. It may be quite possible that you lose weight initially but then, despite the increased effort, results are not phenomenal. One needs to be patient. With sustained performance of *pranayama, bandhas, kriyas* and *asanas,* you will soon attain your ideal body shape and glowing looks.

Surya Namaskar

The technique of solar vitalisation is called *surya namaskar*. In ancient times, *yogis* used to salute Lord Surya by facing the sun and performing this series of movements which is a combination of ten *asanas*. It is usually performed as a warm- up before performing other *asanas*. It is carried out in a cyclic form with the recitation of twelve *mantras* dedicated to Lord Surya. It is advised to chant these *mantras* in each *asana*.

Technique:
- Stand straight with the feet together. Fold your palms in front of your chest. Close your eyes and breathe regularly. Now chant the *mantra, "Om mitraya namaha."*

- Inhale and stretch out your folded palms straight in front of the chest, making them parallel with the floor. Stretch your hands over your head, locking the shoulders and the ears together and stretch backwards. Now chant the *mantra, "Om ravaye namaha."*

- Exhale and bend your body forward till your fingers, palms or hands touch the floor by the side of your feet. Try and touch the knees with your forehead and relax. Now chant the *mantra, "Om suryaya namaha."*

- Inhale and take your right leg back and place both your palms on the floor by the side of your left leg. Stretch your back and arch up as much as possible. Avoid touching the right knee on the floor. Now chant the *mantra, "Om bhanave namaha."*

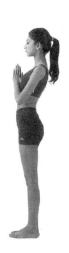
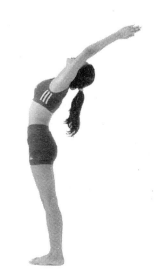
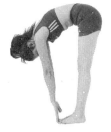
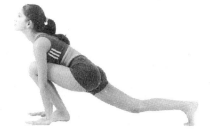

- Exhale and take the right leg backward, making a straight line from the head to the toe. Balance the body weight on the toes and palms. Now chant the *mantra, "Om khagaya namaha."*

- Hold your breath and place your knees on the floor. Now bend your elbows, pressing your chest and forehead on the floor. In this posture, your toes, knees, chest and forehead should touch the floor. Now chant the *mantra, "Om pushnaya namaha."*

- Inhale and stretch your upper body upwards, straightening your elbows and arching the back to look at the sky. Now chant the *mantra, "Om hiranya garbhaya namaha."*

- Exhale and raise your hips upwards as high as possible, tucking the chin inwards towards the chest while looking at the navel. Your heels should remain pressed on the floor. Now chant the *mantra, "Om marichaya namaha."*

- Inhale and bring your left leg forward. Arch your back backwards. Now chant the *mantra, "Om adityaya namaha."*

- Exhale and bring both the legs forward just as in the third posture and touch your toes. Now chant the *mantra, "Om savitre namaha."*

- Inhale and stretch your hands over your head backwards just as in the second posture. Now chant the *mantra, "Om arkaya namaha."*

- Exhale and come back to the first posture. Now chant the mantra, *"Om bhaskaraya namaha."*

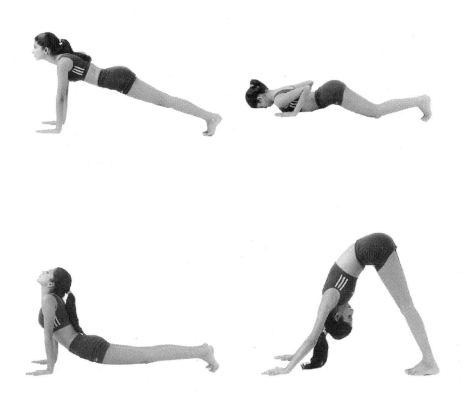

Benefits:

- *Surya namaskar,* being a combination of twelves postures, improves the flexibility of the whole body. If done faster than the normal *yogic* speed, it can improve cardio-respiratory endurance which is an important part of a physical fitness routine.

- It is a wrong notion that Yoga does not reduce weight. If one practices ten cycles of *surya namaskar* to start with and gradually increases this to a hundred cycles, one will definitely lose weight.

- Opens the *granthis* (the physical blockages of the body) and makes the body look young, vibrant and lustrous.

- Improves the auto-immune system of the body, thereby developing resistance to weather. This is apparent when you see *yogis* from the Himalayas roaming around bare-bodied on ice-covered mountains.

- Another benefit is that it balances the vital plexus of our body from the *mooladhar* (the root plexus) to the *brahamarandra* (the crown plexus).

Don'ts:

- People suffering from severe backache or any other spinal problems should consult their physician before performing this *asana.*

- People suffering from severe knee pain should perform these *asanas* very slowly and under expert guidance.

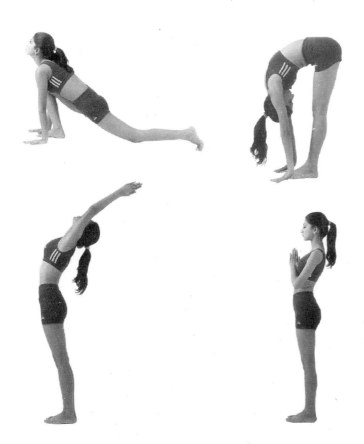

TADASANA

Position:

Take the straight standing posture.

Technique:

- Spread your feet apart by a foot.
- Raise both your hands over the head and hold your palms together.
- Rise upwards on your toes and stretch your whole body up as high as possible.
- Maintain the posture for between thirty seconds to a minute. Keep your breathing as normal as possible throughout the exercise.
- Bring your hands back slowly and exhale. Bring your heels back on the floor and hands to the side of your thighs.

Benefits:

- Helps remove stiffness from the spine and tiredness from the upper part of the body.
- Strengthens the ankles, the smaller joints of the foot and the calf muscles.

Don'ts:

- People suffering from severe ankle pain can perform this posture with their heels on the floor.
- People suffering from Frozen Shoulder should avoid overstretching their arms.

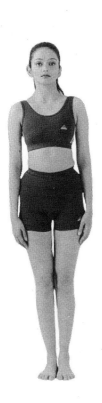
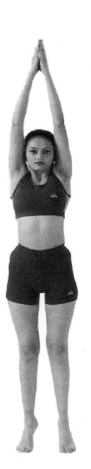

49

ARDHACHAKRASANA

Position:

Take the straight standing posture.

Technique:

- Raise your right hand upto the shoulder level.
- Turn your palm upwards and raise your right hand over the head, stretching it up.
- Exhale and then bend your body to the left side.
- Inhale and come back to the standing posture.
- Repeat the same cycle with the other side.

Benefits:

- Removes fat from the sides of the body.
- Helps get rid of stiff hip joints.
- Helps in curing Asthma. When you bend to a side, one lung gets enlarged while the other gets closed. Shifting the load of two lungs to one clears the blockages in the lungs and improves the functional capacity of the breathing system.

Don'ts:

- Don't bend forward and backwards in this posture.
- Don't hold your breath in this posture.

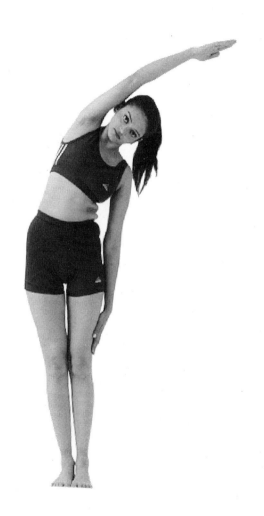

Veerasana

Position:

Take the straight standing posture.

Technique:

- Move your feet apart, keep your hands on the waist and look straight ahead.
- Turn your whole body to the right. Turn the right toes in the same direction.
- Inhale slowly and bend the front knee as much as possible while stretching your body backwards.
- Breathe normally and look up towards the sky.
- Come back to the starting posture and relax.
- Repeat the same cycle on the other side.

Benefits:

- Improves the strength of the back and the knee joints.
- Removes laziness and drowsiness as stretching of the navel region rejuvenates the body.
- Removes postural defects like Sclerosis (rounded back) and keeps the back straight.
- Removes double chin as it stretches the neck backwards.

Don'ts:

- People suffering from backache should perform this *asana* very gently and avoid overstretching backwards.

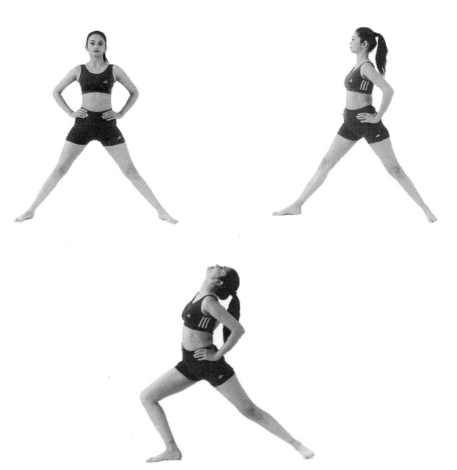

Natrajasana

Position:

Take the straight standing posture.

Technique:

- Spread your feet apart by a foot more than your shoulder width.
- Bend your knees and keep your hands on your thighs. Raise your heels as much as possible and stand on the ball of your feet. Breathe normally.
- Raise your hands over your head and pull your upper body as high as possible. Hold.
- Come back to the starting posture and relax.

Benefits:

- Removes fat from the thighs.
- Brings the calf muscles into shape.
- Strengthens the ankles.
- Removes stiffness from the upper parts of the body.

Don'ts:

- People suffering from severe Arthritis of the knee-joint or those who have had surgery on their knees should consult their doctor before performing this *asana*.

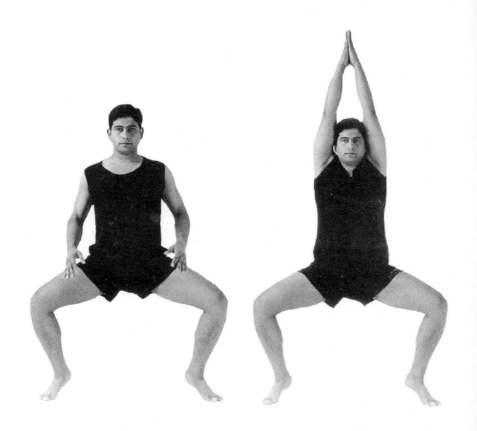

Bakasana

Position:

Take the straight standing posture.

Technique:

- Spread your feet apart and bring them parallel to your shoulders.
- Bend your knees as much as possible and raise your hands up over your head.
- Exhale slowly, bend down and place your palm on the floor. Concenterate on the gap between your palms.
- Rise up slowly.
- Repeat this cycle.

Benefits:

- Stretches your hip muscles, removing the extra flab on the hip.
- Strengthens the knee-joint.
- Stretches the entire back.

Don'ts:

- People suffering from severe knee pain or back problem should avoid this *asana*.

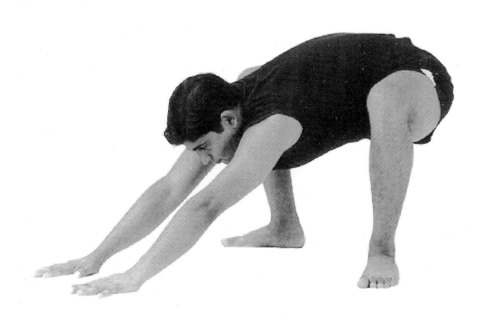

JANUSIRASANA

Position:

Take the long sitting posture.

Technique:

- Bend your right leg and place it so as to touch the inner part of the left thighs. The heel should touch the groin area.
- Slowly raise your hands over your head. Breathe normally.
- Exhale slowly and bend forward. Interlock your fingers and hold your heel.
- Bend forward fully and touch your elbows on the floor. Try and touch your forehead, chest and abdomen on the thighs.
- Breathe normally and maintain the posture for between thirty seconds to one minute.
- Inhale slowly, raise your hands gradually over your head and come back to the long sitting posture.
- Repeat the same cycle on the other side.

Benefits:

- Helps remove stiffness from the spine.
- Stretches calves, hips, thighs, ankles, removing the unwanted flab from all these areas.
- Presses the abdomen, thereby improving digestion.

Don'ts:

- People suffering from lower back pain should avoid this *asana*.

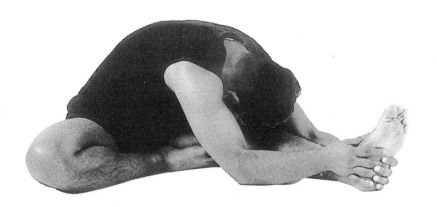

Paschimottanasana

Position:

Take the long sitting posture.

Technique:

- Raise your hands over your head.
- Exhale deeply and bend your body.
- Hold your toes or heels with both your hands and try to pull your body downwards. Try to touch your forehead on your knees.
- Maintain this posture for between thirty seconds to a minute while breathing normally.
- Inhale slowly and raise your hands over your head before returning to the long sitting posture.

Benefits:

- Helps remove stiffness from the spine.
- Stretches calves, hips, thighs, ankles, removing the unwanted flab from all these areas.
- Presses the abdomen, thereby improving digestion.

Don'ts:

- People suffering from lower backache should avoid this *asana*.

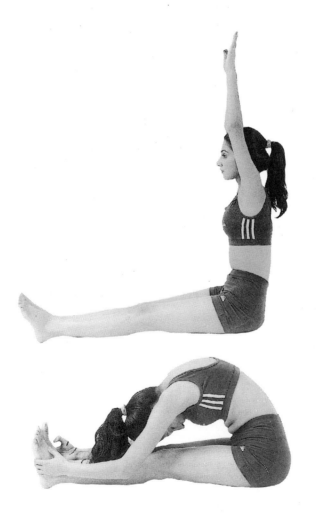

ARDHAKAPOTASANA

Position:

- Take the long sitting posture.

Technique:

- Bend the right leg to bring the knee in front of the body, leaving the left leg behind.
- Place your palms in front and place the front heel away from the groin.
- Inhale slowly and make a cup with your fingertips. Now stretch your upper body backwards and look at the sky.
- Hold this posture for between thirty seconds to a minute.
- Bring your left leg back in front and relax.
- Repeat the same cycle on the other side.

Benefits:

- Stretches the outer portion of the thighs, bringing them into shape.
- Removes double chin.
- Stretches the abdomen thereby removing fat from the abdominal area.
- Strengthens the back muscles.

Don'ts:

- People with severe lower backache and stiff knee-joints should avoid this *asana*.

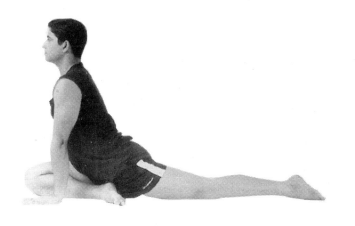

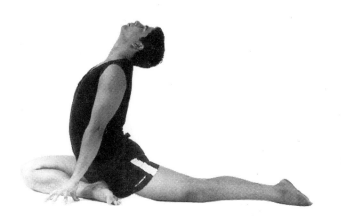

63

TOLUNGASANA

This is an advanced *asana*, hence one should practice the basic version before attempting it.

Position:

Take the posture of *padmasana*.

Technique:

- Place your hands by the side of your hips and raise your hips and crossed legs above the floor.
- Inhale and hold your breath.
- Maintain this posture for between thirty seconds to a minute.
- Exhale and drop your hip and the crossed legs back on the floor slowly.
- Open your crossed legs and go back to the long sitting position.

Benefits:

- Strengthens the entire upper part of the body including the chest, shoulders, forearms and wrists.
- Improves abdominal strength.
- Removes fat from the upper parts of the body.

Don'ts:

- People suffering from Frozen Shoulder, Dislocated Shoulder, or Broken Elbow should avoid this *asana*.

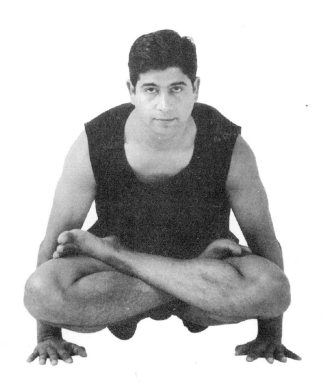

Vajrasana

Position:

Take the long sitting posture.

Technique:

- Bending one leg at the knee bring your foot under the same hip.
- Hold the other foot by the same side hand and place it under the other hip.
- See that the toes do not touch each other and the heels are turned outwards, making a 'V'. You should be sitting on the heels.
- Keep the back straight and place your palms on your knees.
- Breathe normally and maintain this posture for a maximum of two minutes and a minimum of thirty seconds.
- People experiencing pain in the ankles while performing this *asana* may place a pillow each under their hips and ankles so that the pain is minimised. Slowly, after some time, remove the top pillow, later the lower pillow and you will be in *vajrasana*.

Benefits:

- This is the only *asana* which can be performed soon after having a meal as it hastens digestion.
- Helps in increasing the flexibility of ankle-joints.
- Helps in improving the posture.

Don'ts:

- People suffering from severe Arthritis should not attempt this *asana*.
- People who have undergone a knee or spinal surgery should avoid this *asana*.

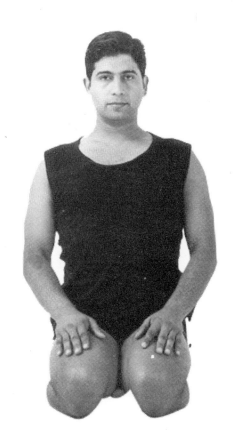

67

Suptavajrasana

Position:

Take the posture of *vajrasana*.

Technique:

- Place your hips between your heels.

- Holding the heels, lean backwards and place your elbows on the floor with the neck stretched backwards. Slowly straighten your elbows and lie down on the floor.
- Try to keep the knees together and place your palms on the thighs.
- Maintain this posture for between thirty seconds to a minute.
- Holding your heels, slowly move upwards placing your elbows on the floor. Press the floor with your palms and slowly return to the sitting posture.
- Bring your legs back to the long sitting posture.

Benefits:

- Stretches the thighs.
- Strengthens the knee-joints and the back muscles.

Don'ts:

- People suffering from knee pain should avoid this *asana*.

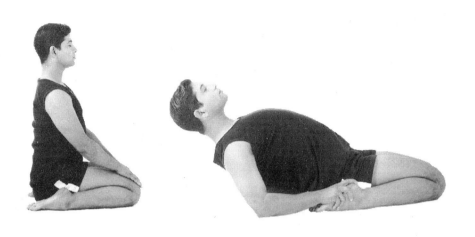

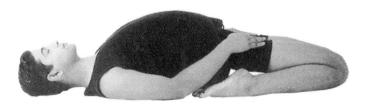

BHUNAMANUTKATASANA

Position:

Take the long sitting posture.

Technique:

- Sit on your heels.
- Put your palms on the cheeks and rest your elbows on the floor.
- Spread your knees and allow the body to bend forward. Bend the elbows, hold the cheeks with your palms and place your face on the floor.
- Slowly stretch your hands and bring them over your head. Now place your forehead on the floor.
- Maintain this posture for between thirty seconds to a minute and exhale deeply.
- Inhale slowly and come back to the long sitting posture.

Benefits:

- Helps to remove fat from the buttocks, thighs and stretches the entire back.
- Improves blood flow to the upper part of the body, removing blockages and stiffness in the upper body.
- Improves the texture of the facial skin.

Don'ts:

- This is an advanced *asana* so only people with high levels of flexibility should attempt it.
- People with severe knee pain should avoid this *asana*.

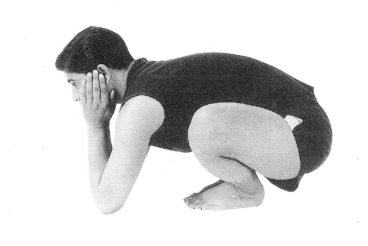

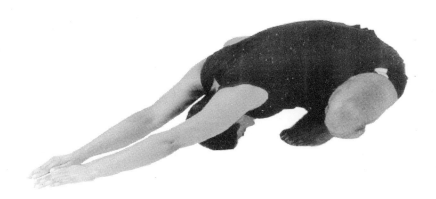

KONASANA

Position:

Take the straight standing posture.

Technique:

- Spread your legs as far apart as possible.
- Exhale and place your palms on the floor, bending your body forward.
- Press the hip away from the mid-line of your body.
- Hold this posture and breathe normally for between thirty seconds to a minute.
- Moving the heels and the toes inward and upward from both the sides, bring your heels together. Inhale and stand up.

Benefits:

- Increases strength of the arms.
- Stretches the inner part of the thighs and helps tone them.
- Stretches the hip, hamstring and the calf besides removing fat from these areas.

Don'ts:

- People suffering from severe low backache should avoid this *asana*.

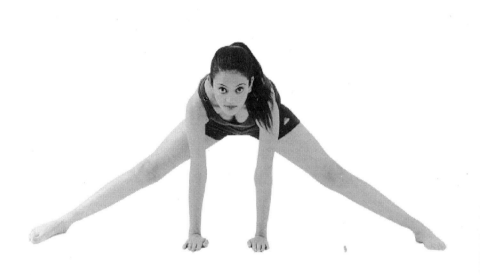

Ekpad Pavanmuktasana

Position:

Lie on the back and place your hands by the side of your thighs.

Technique:

- Interlock your fingers, bend your right knee and place your interlocked hands over the knee. Exhale slowly, pulling your knee towards your chest.
- Pull your upper body and touch the chin on your knees.
- Maintain this posture for between thirty seconds to a minute and breathe normally.
- Relax your grip, straighten your leg and come back to the supine lying posture.
- Repeat the same cycle on the other side.

Benefits:

- Removes lower backache or stiffness from the lumbar area of the back.
- Stretches the hamstring and the hips, removing extra fat from these areas.
- Improves flexibility of the hip joint and the knee joint.
- Removes unwanted gas from the body and thus the flatulence.

Don'ts:

- People suffering from Cervical Spondylosis should not raise their body up and bring it over the chin, they should keep their head on the floor.

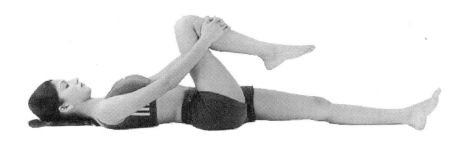

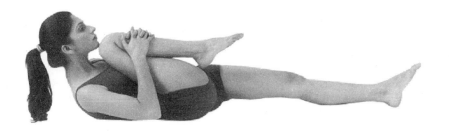

Sampurna Pavanmuktasana

Position:

Lie flat on the floor with the hands by the side of your thighs.

Technique:

- Bend both your knees.
- Interlock your fingers and bring the hands over your knees.
- Pull your knees towards the chest.
- Breathe normally, then slowly exhale and bring your chin over your knees.
- Maintain this posture for thirty seconds to a minute and breathe normally.
- Slowly release your hands and return to the supine lying posture.

Benefits:

- Removes lower backache and stiffness from the lumbar area of the back.
- Stretches the hamstring and the hips, removing extra fat from these areas.
- Improves flexibility of the hip joint and the knee joint.
- Removes unwanted gas from the body.

Don'ts:

- People suffering from Cervical Spondylosis should not raise their upper body. They should keep their head on the floor.

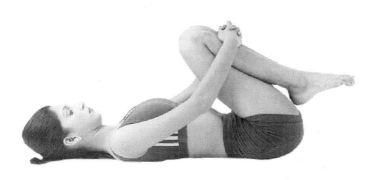

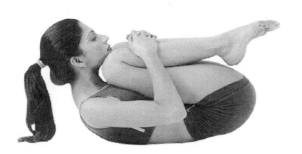

Supta Ekpad Uttanasana

Position:

Lie flat on the floor with the hands by the side of your thighs.

Technique:

- Bend your knee and hold the toe of your right foot with both your hands as shown.
- Raise your upper body, exhale and straighten the knee joint slowly till your legs are straight. Keep your left leg straight, stretching the toes downwards.
- Maintain this posture for between thirty seconds to one minute.
- Slowly release your hold and come back to the supine lying posture.
- Repeat the same cycle on the other side.

Benefits:

- Removes fat from the hips, thigh and the calf region.
- Stretches the upper back removing stiffness from the area.

Don'ts:

- People with a stiff knee should straighten their knees slowly, else it may lead to a muscle injury.

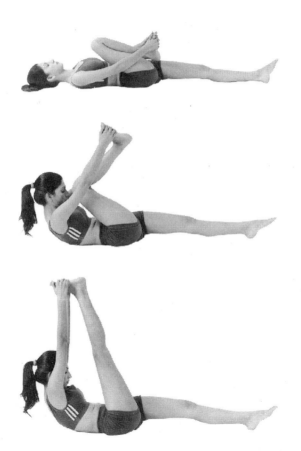

Santolanasana

Position:

Lie flat on your stomach with your hands by the side and your chin on the floor. Your toes should be tucked inwards.

Technique:

- Bring your hands to the side of the chest.
- Raise your entire body by straightening the arms and doing a push-up.
- Keeping your body straight, stretch your body ahead and shift your weight on the upper part of your body.
- Maintain this posture for between thirty seconds to a minute and breathe normally.
- Place your knee on the floor, relax your hands and sit on your heels.
- Straighten your legs and return to the long sitting posture.

Benefits:

- Helps to tone up the muscles and remove extra fat from the arms and the shoulder region.
- Strengthens the chest area and gives it a definite shape.
- Strengthens the muscles on the sides of the body and gives you a nice 'V' shape.

Don'ts:

- People suffering from Tennis Elbow and wrist and elbow problems should avoid this *asana*.

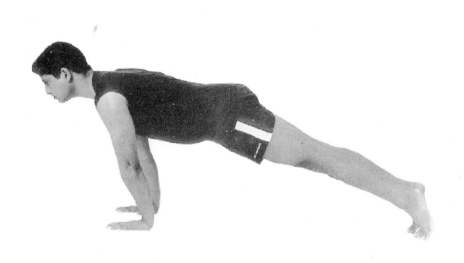

BHUNAMAN KAKASANA

Position:

Lie flat on the stomach, chin touching the floor and hands by the side; your toes should be tucked inwards.

Technique:

- Bring your hands by the side of your chest. Raise your entire body by straightening your arms and doing a press-up.
- Place your left knee on the floor and raise your right leg up. Bend your elbows and go down towards the floor without touching it.
- Maintain this posture for between thirty seconds to a minute, breathing normally.
- Bring your leg down and place your chest on the floor. Now, lie down on your stomach and relax.
- Repeat the same cycle on the other side.

Benefits:

- Improves the strength of the upper parts of the body.
- Improves wrist strength and tones the muscles of the arms, biceps and triceps.

Don'ts:

- People suffering from Tennis Elbow and wrist and elbow problems should avoid this *asana*.

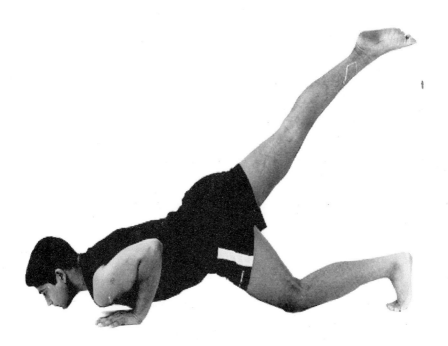

Sahaj Vyagrasana

Position:

Take the dog posture where you rest on your knees and hands as shown.

Technique:

- Look straight ahead and pull your neck upwards.
- Stretch one of your legs straight and then inhale slowly while raising your leg as high as possible. Keep both the toes stretched.
- Tighten the hip muscles and maintain this posture for between thirty seconds to a minute.
- Bring your knee back on the floor and relax.
- Repeat the same cycle with the other leg.

Benefits:

- Tones the hip muscles and removes extra fat from the hips.
- Strengthens the neck and back muscles.

Don'ts:

- This *asana* should not be performed on a hard surface as it might hurt the knee joints.

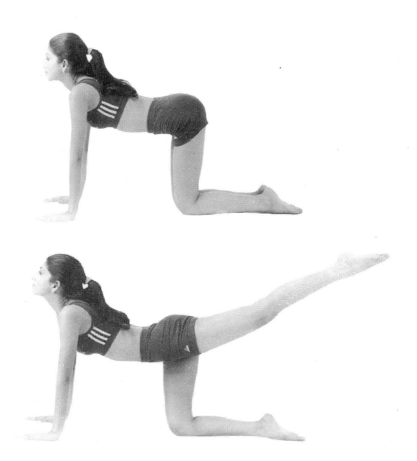

85

Purna Vyagrasana

Position:

Take the dog posture.

Technique:

- Look straight ahead, raise one leg straight up and parallel to the floor.
- Inhale and bend the knee of the raised leg. Then slowly raise the knee as high as possible. Contract the hamstring and hip muscles as tight as possible.
- Maintain this posture for between thirty seconds to a minute and exhale deeply.
- Come back to the starting posture.
- Repeat the same cycle with the other leg.

Benefits:

- In addition to the benefits of *sahaj vaygrasana*, this *asana* also helps to improve the back thigh muscles and the hip muscles.

Don'ts:

- This *asana* should not be performed on a hard surface as it might hurt the knee joint.

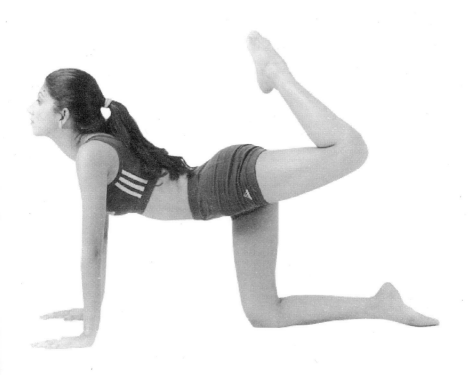

Asanas for the Abdomen

Sahaj Ubhay Padang Utthitasana

Position:

Take the long sitting posture.

Technique:

- Take your hands away from the hip. Bend your knees and place the heels a foot away from the hip.
- Drop your elbows on the floor and stretch your legs ahead, raising them to an angle of 45° above the floor.
- Inhale and hold your breath in this posture as long as you can.
- Exhale and lie down on your back. Go back to the long sitting posture.

Benefits:

- Strengthens and removes fat from the middle and upper abdominal area.

Don'ts:

- People suffering from lower backache should raise one leg instead of both.
- People suffering from Cervical Spondylosis should keep their neck straight to avoid excessive strain.

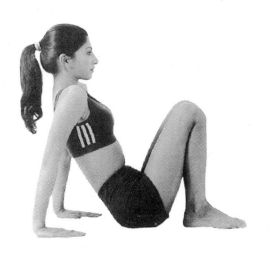

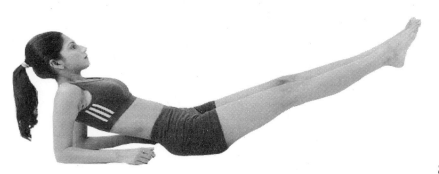

89

Sampurna Ubhay Padang Utthitasana

Position:

Take the long sitting posture.

Technique:

- Stretch your hands behind your hips.
- Bend your knees and place them a foot away from the hip. Look straight ahead.
- Bend your elbows and place them on the floor; raise both the legs together to 90° above the ground keeping your toes stretched upwards.
- Inhale and maintain the posture as long as you can hold your breath.
- Exhale slowly. Relax and place your legs on the floor. Lie down on your back.

Benefits:

- Helps to remove fat as well as strengthen and tone the lower abdominal area.

Don'ts:

- People suffering from lower backache and upper backache should come down with their knees bent to avoid straining the lower back.

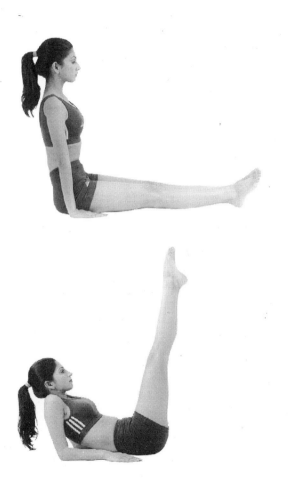

Naukasana

Position:

Lie down flat on the back, with your hands on the thighs.

Technique:

- Exhale slowly and raise your upper and lower body upwards together to take the form of a boat.
- Maintain this posture for as long as you can hold your breath.
- Bring your back and legs back on the floor. Then inhale deeply and relax.

Benefits:

- Helps strengthen the entire abdominal area — from the upper to the lower abdomen.

Don'ts:

- Keep your neck straight and don't tuck your chin on the chest.
- Make sure that you exhale while coming up (into the posture).

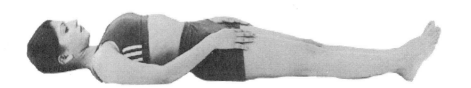

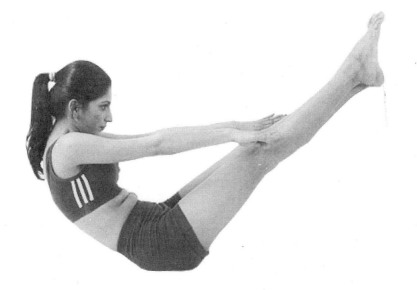

93

Uttana Hasta Merudandasana

Position:

Lie flat on your back with your hands by the side of your thighs.

Technique:
- Bend your knees and place your heels one foot away from the hip.
- Exhale and then slowly raise your upper body while turning to one side.
- Maintain this posture for as long as you can hold your breath.
- Relax and come back to the long sitting posture.
- Repeat on the other side.

Benefits:
- Strengthens the muscles present on the sides of the abdomen.

Don'ts:
- Change postures very slowly and avoid sudden movements.
- Be aware of the stretching in your spine. Do not overstrain.

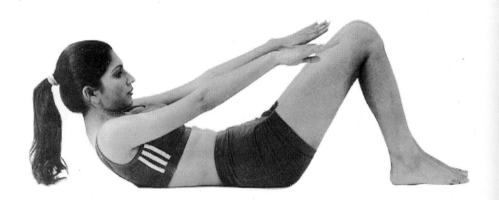

Saral Hasta Bhujangasana

Position:

Lie on your stomach with your chin touching the ground and the palms resting face down next to your thighs.

Technique:

- Bring your palms next to your shoulders.
- Stretch your upper body upwards, straightening your elbows and arching the back to look towards the sky.
- Maintain this posture for thirty seconds.

Benefits:

- Helps remove stiffness from the front part of the body including the chest, shoulders and neck.
- Stretches the abdominal muscles and helps remove flab from this area.
- Helps to cure many urino-genital problems for men and gynaecological problems for women.
- Removes lower back pain by strengthening the muscles of the back.

Don'ts:

- This *asana* should be performed after completing the set of abdomen-specific *asanas* so that the abdominal muscles stretch and do not become stiff and painful.
- People suffering from Hernia, Hydrocil or those who have undergone stomach surgery should avoid this *asana*.
- People with severe backache or spinal injury should consult their doctor before attempting this *asana*.

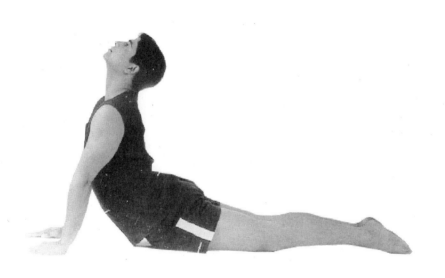

8

Diet

Diet is an important aspect of weight reduction since it is the diet that regulates the calorie intake. But before we discuss the kind of food we should eat, let us understand what food is actually made up of and how different nutrients play different roles in functioning of the human body.

Food is made up of different nutrients. Macronutrients generally provide energy and are needed in large quantities; micronutrients are needed in small quantities and are not a source of energy.

Macronutrients

Macronutrients are the basic nutrients that the body requires. These are:

Proteins

Proteins are made up of amino acids which are the building blocks for muscle tissue, organs, skin, bones and tendons to some extent. They help to build, repair and maintain muscle tissues. However, while consuming protein-rich foods, it is important to know that not all proteins are usable by the body. Eggs, meat and fish contain proteins that are complete but foods like milk, cheese, rice, soybean, potato, wheat and beans have percentages of incomplete proteins. Vegetarians must combine food to provide complete proteins to the body. Cereals and milk, whole wheat bread and cheese, rice and beans, rice and dal (lentils), wheat bread and beans are combinations that give the body a complete protein-rich diet.

Carbohydrates

Carbohydrates are composed of simple or complex sugar and starch molecules. They provide the fuel or energy required by the body and are the easiest form of foods that the body can convert into energy. The basic categories of carbohydrates are:

Monosaccharides
>   Glucose (blood sugar)
>   Fructose (fruit sugar)
>   Galactose (a kind of milk sugar)

Oligosaccharides
>   Sucrose (table sugar)
>   Lactose (milk sugar)
>   Maltose (malt sugar)

Polysaccharides
>   Plant polysaccharides
>   Animal polysaccharides (glycogen)

As carbohydrates get more complex, it becomes more difficult for the body to break them down. Simple carbohydrates like fructose are quickly converted into energy, whereas complex carbohydrates (starchy foods like rice and potato) release energy slowly over a period of time. Several weight-loss diets cut down severely on all carbohydrates making the person weak and unhealthy. A good diet should cut down on 'bad' carbohydrates like refined wheat (pastries, white bread, maida) and sugars. Whole wheat products can be consumed in moderation. Even starchy foods like rice and potatoes can be eaten to a lesser degree but not in combination with fat (butter or oil) which can lead to weight gain.

Fats

Fats are nutrients that contain the highest concentration of calories. They preserve the body's heat, cushion and protect the major organs and constitute the largest source of stored energy in the body. While exercising, more and more fat gets burnt as you spend more and more time on exercising. The last few minutes of your exercise will burn more fat than the first few minutes. Fat molecules are either saturated, unsaturated or polyunsaturated. Meat, poultry, eggs, milk products and chocolate contain large amounts of saturated fat. Unsaturated fats are found in olive oil, peanut oil, avocado and cashew nuts. Polyunsaturated fats are found in foods like walnuts, sunflower oil, corn oil, fish and safflower oil. Fats are the enemies of obese people and should be consumed in very small quantities. One should try and eat less of saturated fats and more of polyunsaturated and unsaturated fats because the more saturated the fat is, the more likely it is to stay in your body, adding to your body weight and clogging your arteries.

Water

Water is also considered a basic nutrient as it is required by the body in large quantities. It is obviously not a source of energy but needs to be consumed regularly so that the entire system is literally kept 'flushed'. Water is the medium by which chemicals can be transported and reactions among the various nutrients can take place.

Micronutrients

Other nutrients that the body uses in very small quantities are called micronutrients. They include:

Vitamins

Vitamins are organic substances that act as catalysts for important reactions taking place in the body. They neither add to body weight nor do they supply energy to the body. Vitamins can be divided into two categories: water-soluble and fat-soluble. Water-soluble vitamins are not stored in the body and excess amounts are removed through the urine; fat-soluble vitamins are stored in the fatty tissues of the body.

Water-soluble vitamins

B1   (thiamin)
B2   (riboflavin)
B3   (niacin, nicotinic acid, nicotinamide)
B5   (pantothenic acid)
B6   (pyridoxine)
B12 (cyanobalamin)

Biotin
Folate (folic acid, folacin)
Vitamin C (ascorbic acid)
Vitamin A (retinol)

Fat-soluble vitamins
Vitamin A
Vitamin D
Vitamin E
Vitamin K

All the vitamins play a vital role in the smooth functioning of the body. Since fat-soluble vitamins can be stored in the body, they need to be consumed less often. Water-soluble vitamins need to be taken on a daily basis. Make sure that you eat enough foods containing all these vitamins. Green leafy vegetables, nuts, milk, whole grain, beans, dried fruit, sunflower seeds, berries, melons and citrus fruits are all good sources of vitamins.

Minerals

Minerals are inorganic substances that are needed for many bodily functions. There are twenty-two metallic elements in the body and they make up four per cent of the body weight, besides playing a role in many metabolic processes and helping in the synthesis of glycogen, proteins and fats. The important minerals that the body requires are calcium, phosphorus, magnesium, potassium, sodium, sulphur and chlorine. These are found in plants and meat and the body requires very small quantities of them. Other minerals like iron are also important but are required in still smaller amounts. As long as you take a balanced diet, you can generally count on getting enough minerals.

Energy Content of Food

Every reaction that takes place in the human body requires energy. The amount of energy contained in a certain amount of food is measured in calories. A calorie actually refers to the amount of heat given off in the oxidation process that occurs inside every cell. Fire, for example, is a kind of rapid oxidation where heat is given off. In the same way, a slower process happens inside every cell.

All the macronutrients — proteins, carbohydrates and fat – are a source of energy and therefore, contain calories. However, 1 gram of protein contains 4 calories whereas 1 gram of fat contains 9 calories. Those who want to lose weight should minimise their fat consumption. Eating large amounts of carbohydrates results in the same intake of calories and is of no use as excess calories will end up being stored in the body as fat anyway.

Yoga and Diet

Yogis divide food into three groups — *satvic*, *tamasic* and *rajasic*. *Satvic* food includes whole grains, fresh vegetables, fruits, milk, curd, nuts, legumes, sprouts and herbs. *Tamasic* food includes all frozen and fried foods, polished and refined grains, alcohol, meat and fungus like mushrooms that grow on decayed matter. *Rajasic* food includes sweets, caffeine, onions, garlic and spices. Yoga recommends a basically *satvic* diet that is rich in whole grains, fibrous vegetables and fruits, and is low in fat content. *Tamasic* food should be completely avoided and *rajasic* food can be consumed occasionally. Meat of all kinds, including fish, should be avoided. One should consume whole wheat as opposed to refined wheat which is not easy to digest. Sprouted foods are also prescribed as they have plenty of vitamins and minerals which give strength to the body and keep the skin glowing. Avoid all tinned, processed and refined foods. Water is a very important nutrient according to the *yogis*. A person should consume at least fifteen glasses of water every day to remove the toxins of the body through urine. Water also decreases the food's acidic levels and prevents the food from getting completely broken down into calories.

My recommendation to anyone, especially those trying to lose weight, is that the most important thing is to maintain a balanced diet without depriving yourself of the foods you enjoy. Deprivation will only lead to overeating later on. Instead, enjoy all kinds of food but remember to eat them in the right quantities and the right combination. Starch when taken with fats or proteins makes a lethal combination. Starch increases the level of insulin which is the fat regulating hormone in your body. If you eat fat and starch at the same time, the fat immediately gets stored away in your fat cells. Avoid combinations like bread and butter, French fries and potato chips which are very fattening. Starch eaten along with proteins will also result in the body storing fat. Proteins further enhance the effect that starch has on insulin. So combinations like white bread and cheese (pizza), eggs and bread, potatoes and meat, hamburgers (meat and bread) are the worst combinations as they combine protein/fat with starch. Even vegetarian foods that are rich in proteins like milk, cheese, peanuts and soya-bean, usually contain fat, though in a lesser percentage. Try to eat starchy foods separately with vegetables and eat proteins and fats along with vegetables to avoid unnecessary storage of fat. When eating snacks, try to have fruits, roasted chick peas (chana), sprouted beans or whole wheat crackers. If you want to lose weight, cut out sugar and saturated fats completely from your diet. Instead of sugar, use a little bit of honey as a sweetener. When you eat vegetables, try to steam them instead of frying or boiling them as it helps preserve the nutrients in them. Cut out vegetable oil and use sunflower or olive oil, as they are richer in unsaturated fats and polyunsaturated fats.

People living along Mediterranean coast have one of the healthiest diets in the world. They have lower rates of obesity and hence fewer cases of high blood pressure and heart disease. A healthy balanced meal has become a part of people's lifestyle here. Typically, Mediterranean people (those from southern Italy, France, Spain, Morocco and Libya) use plenty of olive oil in their cooking, eat plenty of cereals (principally bread), pulses, legumes, nuts, vegetables, fruits and to a lesser degree, cheese, milk, eggs, fish and a little red wine with every meal. Bread is never eaten with butter, and sweets and most meat dishes are eaten on rare occasions quite unlike India. If you enjoy a drink once in a while, drink red wine as it contains fewer calories and has shown in certain cases to aid the digestive process.

Food should be enjoyed, but not indulged in. If you eat all kinds of food in moderation along with the practice of Yoga, there is no reason for you to gain weight.

But if you want to lose weight effectively and rapidly, I will suggest two kinds of diets: the first is a very low-calorie diet where you reduce weight rapidly; and the second is a balanced diet that you can shift to when you want to maintain your weight.

Low Calorie Diet

8:00 a.m. — Start the day with a few fruits (no bananas) and some tea or coffee with milk (but no sugar).

12 noon — Have a large vegetable salad containing chick peas (chana) or sprouts.

1:30 p.m. — Have a soup, steamed vegetables and some paneer (cottage cheese) or one cup of dal.

4:00 p.m. — Eat two whole-wheat biscuits and some tea or coffee with no milk or sugar.

8:00 p.m. — Have salad, plenty of green vegetables and two chapattis (or two slices of whole-wheat bread.)

Balanced Diet

8:00 a.m. — Start the day with a few fruits (no bananas) and a bowl of cereal and low-fat (skimmed) milk. You can have tea or coffee with milk but no sugar.

12 noon — Have a large helping of vegetable salad containing cottage cheese (paneer), chick peas (chana) or sprouts.

2:00 p.m. — Have a soup, steamed vegetables and two chapattis.

5:00 p.m. — Eat two whole-wheat biscuits and some tea or coffee with milk but no sugar.

107

8:00 p.m. —   End the day with salad, plenty of vegetables (steamed or lightly sauteed in olive oil) and two chapattis (or two slices of whole wheat bread).

You can follow the first diet for as long as 10 days, after which you can switch to the balanced diet. Follow this diet for about 20 days, as it gives your body a resting period, after which you can resume the low-calorie diet. This way your body has some time to adjust to its new weight and you don't feel the urge to overeat and regain your lost weight. After you have reached your optimal weight, continue with the balanced diet and make it a part of your lifestyle. Feel free to adapt it to your palate, keeping in mind the basic guidelines of healthy eating as mentioned in this chapter.

Losing weight is not impossible, no matter how overweight you are. It is a simple matter of making a decision within yourself and then changing your habits by introducing Yoga and good wholesome food in your daily life. Once you begin the practice of Yoga, it will be virtually impossible for you to gain weight again.